PLANT BASED MILK; Health benefits and formulation

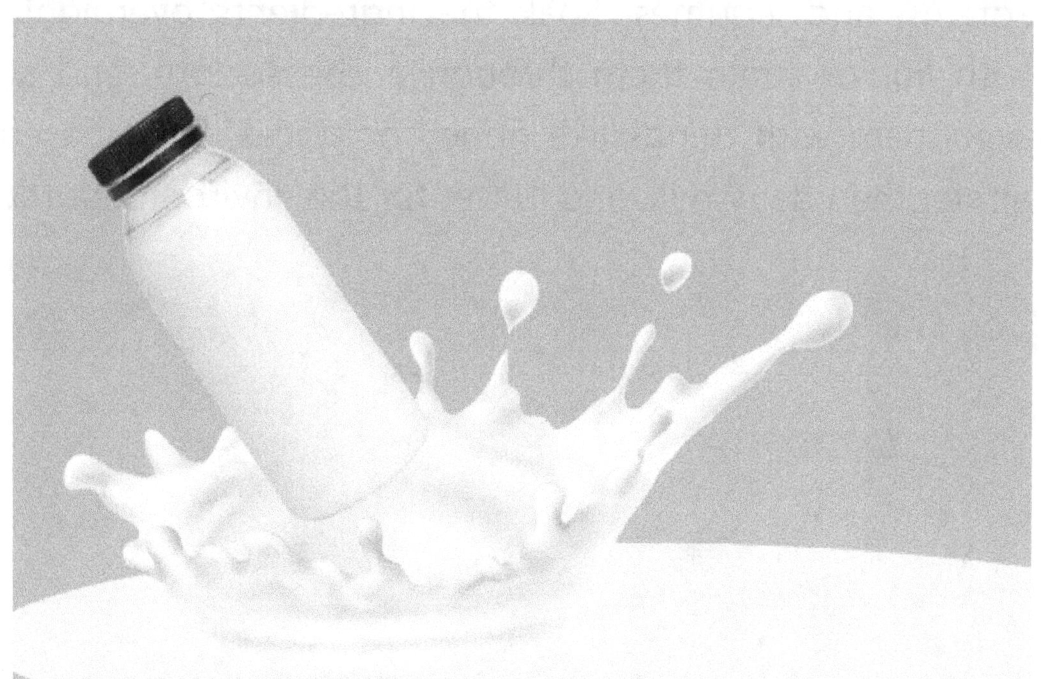

Olabimtan Olabode.H

Synopsis

Making plant-based milk is a great way to have a tasty and nutritious alternative to dairy milk. You can choose different types of plant-based milk, like almond milk or oat milk.

You will need to soak the plant-based ingredients in water and blend them together with water. Then strain the milk to make it creamy and smooth. Plant-based milk is a fun way to mix up your diet and help the environment.

You can make plant-based milks at home using ingredients like nuts, seeds, grains, and legumes. Soak the ingredients overnight, blend them with liquid, strain them through a cheesecloth, and sweeten and flavor them with things like honey or spices. Plant-based milks are healthier than dairy milk and better for the environment too.

Table of Contents

ISBN: 9798864172742

Cover design by: Art Painter

Library of Congress Control Number: 2018675309

Printed in the United States of America

Chapter One.
Introduction to Plant-Based Milk

Plant-based milk is a great alternative to traditional dairy milk for those looking for a healthier and more sustainable option. Plant-based milk is made from a variety of plant sources, such as almonds, oats, soy, rice, and coconut. It is a great way to get more plant-based proteins, vitamins, minerals, and other nutrients into your diet.

 The milk is completely free of cholesterol, making it an ideal choice for those with heart health concerns.

In addition, plant-based milk is free of lactose, making it a great choice for those who are lactose intolerant.

Plant-based milk is also lower in calories and fat than traditional dairy milk, making it a great choice for those looking to lose weight or maintain a healthy diet.

Plant-based milk is now available in a variety of forms, including powders, creams, and ready-to-drink varieties. The powdered form of plant-based milk is easy to store and is shelf-stable for long periods of time.

Making your own plant-based milk at home with a powdered form is also very easy to do and is a great way to save money. Simply add the desired amount of powder to water and stir until fully dissolved.

This process can be done in a matter of minutes and the resulting plant-based milk will have a creamy and delicious taste.

The health benefits of plant-based powdered milk are numerous as it is rich in plant-based proteins, vitamins, minerals, and other nutrients. It is also free of cholesterol and lactose, making it a great choice for those with heart health concerns or who are lactose intolerant.

Plant-based powdered milk is also lower in calories and fat than traditional dairy milk, making it a great choice for those looking to lose weight or maintain a healthy diet.
Finally, making your own plant-based milk at home with a powdered form is both easy and cost-effective.

Chapter Two
Nutritional Benefits of Plant-Based Milk

Powder-based plant milks can provide significant health benefits due to their nutrient content. Plant-based milks are naturally high in essential vitamins and minerals, including iron, zinc, magnesium, and vitamins A, B, and D. In comparison to dairy milk, these milks are also lower in saturated fat and cholesterol and this makes them a great option for those looking to reduce their intake of animal products, while still getting the benefits of a nutritious drink.

Plant-based milks also provide a great source of plant-based proteins. Many varieties contain up to 8 grams of protein per serving, which is comparable to the amount of protein found in dairy milk. This makes them a great option for those looking to build or maintain muscle mass. Additionally, since protein helps the body absorb and utilize other essential vitamins and minerals, it's important to make sure you're getting enough of it in your diet. Plant-based milks are also a great source of dietary fiber. Unlike dairy milk, plant-based milks contain no lactose, which makes them easier to digest for those who are lactose intolerant. Additionally, the dietary fiber found in plant-based milks is beneficial for promoting a healthy digestive system. In addition to their nutritional benefits, plant-based milks are also much better for the environment than dairy milk. The production of dairy milk requires large amounts of land, water, and energy, which can be detrimental to the environment.

By contrast, the production of plant-based milks requires significantly less land and energy, making them a much more sustainable option. Generally, plant-based milks are a great option for those looking to get the nutritional benefits of a dairy milk alternative, while also reducing their environmental impact. With their high protein, fiber, and vitamin content, these milks can provide a nutritious, delicious, and sustainable option for anyone looking to improve their health.

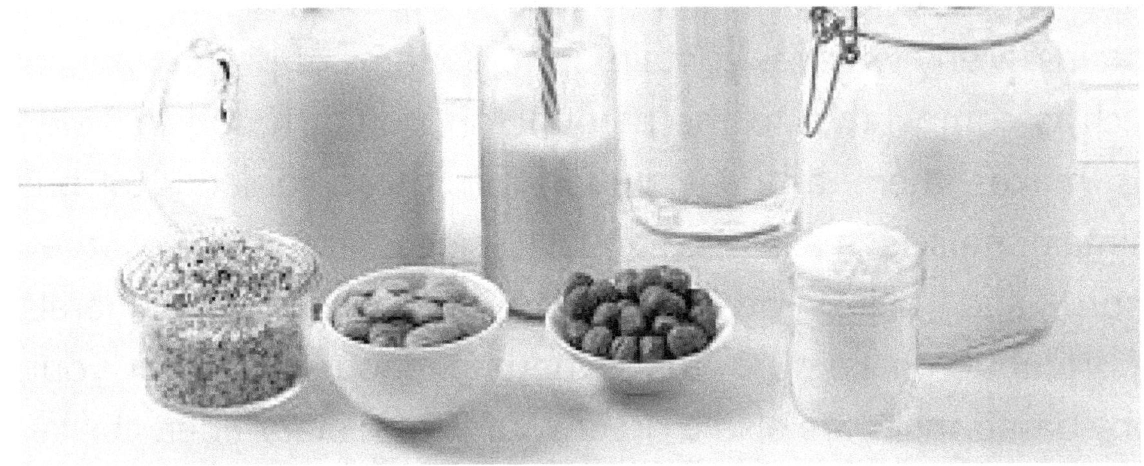

Chapter Three
Health Benefits of Plant-Based Powdered Milk

Plant-based powdered milk is becoming increasingly popular among health-conscious individuals due to its many health benefits. Plant-based powdered milk is a type of plant-based milk that has been dried and milled into a fine powder. It can be reconstituted with water and used in a variety of recipes, from smoothies to baked goods. Plant-based powdered milk is a great source of essential vitamins and minerals. It is a good source of calcium, iron, magnesium, and vitamin B12. It also contains a variety of essential fatty acids, including omega-3 fatty acids.

These essential nutrients are important for maintaining proper bone health, cardiovascular health, and blood sugar levels.

Plant-based powdered milk is also low in saturated fat and sugar, making it a great choice for those looking to maintain a healthy weight. It is also rich in antioxidants and other phytonutrients that help to protect the body from the damaging effects of free radicals. This can help to reduce the risk of developing certain forms of cancer, as well as other chronic diseases. Additionally, plant-based powdered milk is high in fiber, which can help to support digestive health and prevent constipation.

Plant-based powdered milk is also an excellent source of plant-based protein as protein is very essential for the growth and repair of the body's tissues, as well as for maintaining healthy muscles. Plant-based proteins are also easier to digest than animal proteins, making them a great choice for those looking to boost their protein intake.

Finally, plant-based powdered milk is a great choice for those who are lactose intolerant. It is free of lactose, making it an ideal choice for those who are unable to digest dairy products.

It is a vegan-friendly option, as it does not contain any animal products. Generally, plant-based powdered milk is an excellent choice for those looking to improve their overall health. It is an excellent source of essential vitamins and minerals, as well as antioxidants and other phytonutrients. Also, it is a great source of plant-based protein, and is free of lactose, making it a great choice for those who are lactose intolerant. Finally, it is an affordable and convenient option, making it an ideal choice for those looking to make healthy dietary changes.

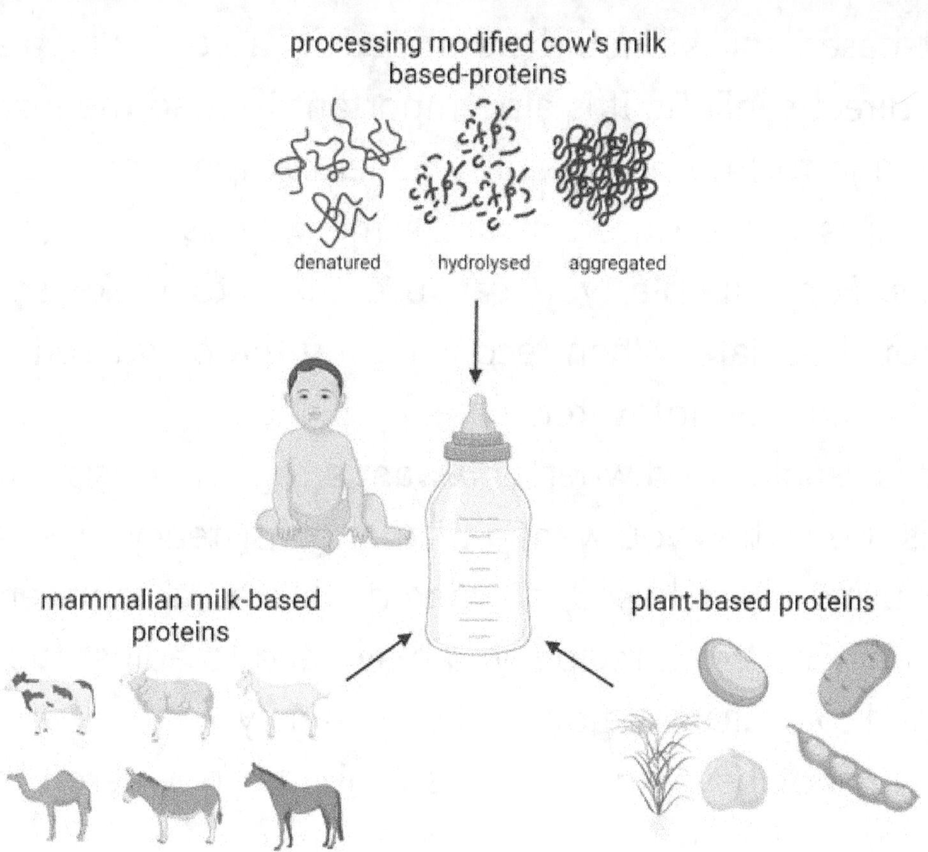

Chapter Four

How to Use Plant-Based Powdered Milk

Plant-based powdered milk has become increasingly popular in recent years as people become more health conscious. Plant-based powdered milks are made from plant sources such as soy, almonds, coconut, and oats. They are a great alternative to traditional dairy-based powdered milks, as they are low in saturated fat and cholesterol, and are typically non-dairy and lactose-free.

Plant-based milks also contain more vitamins, minerals, and antioxidants than traditional dairy milks. When it comes to using plant-based powdered milk, there are a few things to keep in mind.

First, plant-based milks should be stored in a cool, dry place, and away from direct sunlight. It is also important to read the instructions on the package for the best results. Generally speaking, plant-based powdered milks can be used in the same way as traditional dairy-based milks. For example, you can use them to make smoothies, lattes, or hot chocolate. When reconstituting the powdered milk, you can use either cold or hot water.

Cold water is usually used when you want a thicker consistency, while hot water is used when you want a thinner consistency.

If you are using plant-based powdered milk as a replacement for traditional dairy milk in a recipe, you may need to adjust the amount of liquid used to achieve the desired consistency.

When making hot beverages, you can mix the powdered milk with the other ingredients and then heat the mixture.

Alternatively, you can mix the powdered milk with hot water before adding the other ingredients.

It is important to note that some plant-based milks may not foam or froth as much as traditional dairy milks, so you may need to adjust the recipe accordingly. Plant-based powdered milk is a great alternative to traditional dairy-based milks. It is low in saturated fat and cholesterol and is generally non-dairy and lactose-free.

It is important to read the instructions on the package for the best results when using plant-based powdered milk. It can be used in the same way as traditional dairy-based milks, although you may need to adjust the amount of liquid used to achieve the desired consistency.

When making hot beverages, you may need to adjust the recipe accordingly to account for the fact that some plant-based milks may not foam or froth as much as traditional dairy milks.

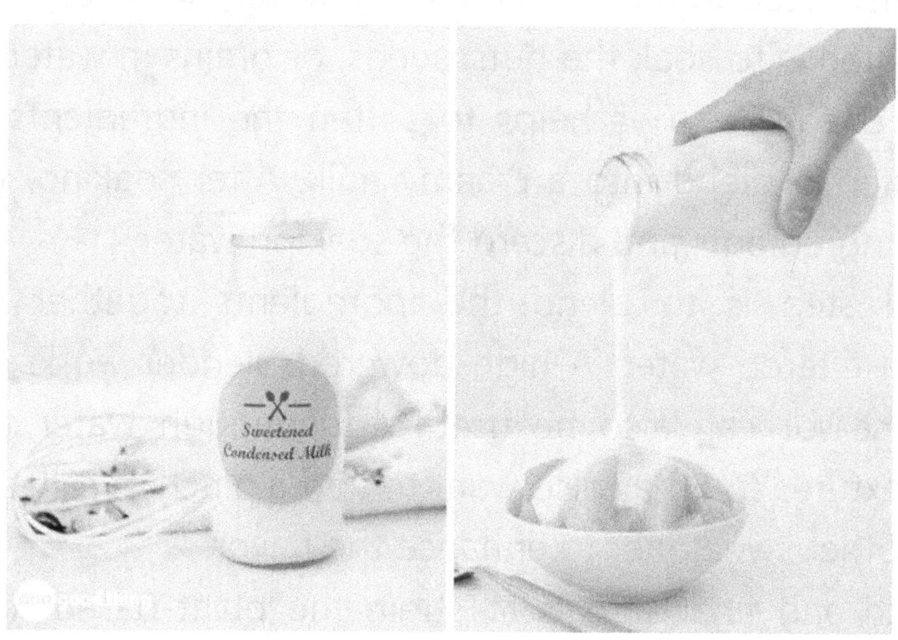

Chapter Five

Process Overview of Plant-Based Milk

Making plant-based milk is an easy process that requires few ingredients and minimal effort. Plant-based milk is a great alternative to dairy milk, and it can be made from a variety of sources such as nuts, oats, and seeds.

The process of making plant-based milk is simple and can be done in just a few steps. Here is a step-by-step guide to making your own plant-based milk.

The first step in making plant-based milk is to gather the necessary ingredients. Depending on the type of plant-based milk you are making, you will need to choose the right type of nut, seed, or grain. Popular options include almonds, cashews, oats, and hemp seeds. You will also need to have some filtered water on hand.

The next step is to soak the nuts, seeds, or grains in water for several hours or overnight. This helps to soften the ingredients and make them easier to blend into a creamy milk. After soaking, you should rinse the ingredients and discard the soaking water.

The third step is to blend the ingredients together with some additional filtered water. A high-powered blender works best, but a food processor can also be used. Add enough water to create a creamy texture. You may also want to add a pinch of salt, a few dates, or some other sweetener to enhance the flavor.

The fourth and final step is to strain the plant-based milk using a cheesecloth or a fine-mesh strainer. This helps to remove any pieces of nuts, seeds, or grains that did not blend completely and gives the milk a smoother texture.

Once strained, the milk is ready to be enjoyed. Making plant-based milk is a fun and easy process that can be done in a few simple steps.

With just a few ingredients and minimal effort, you can make a delicious and nutritious plant-based milk that is perfect for adding to your favorite recipes.

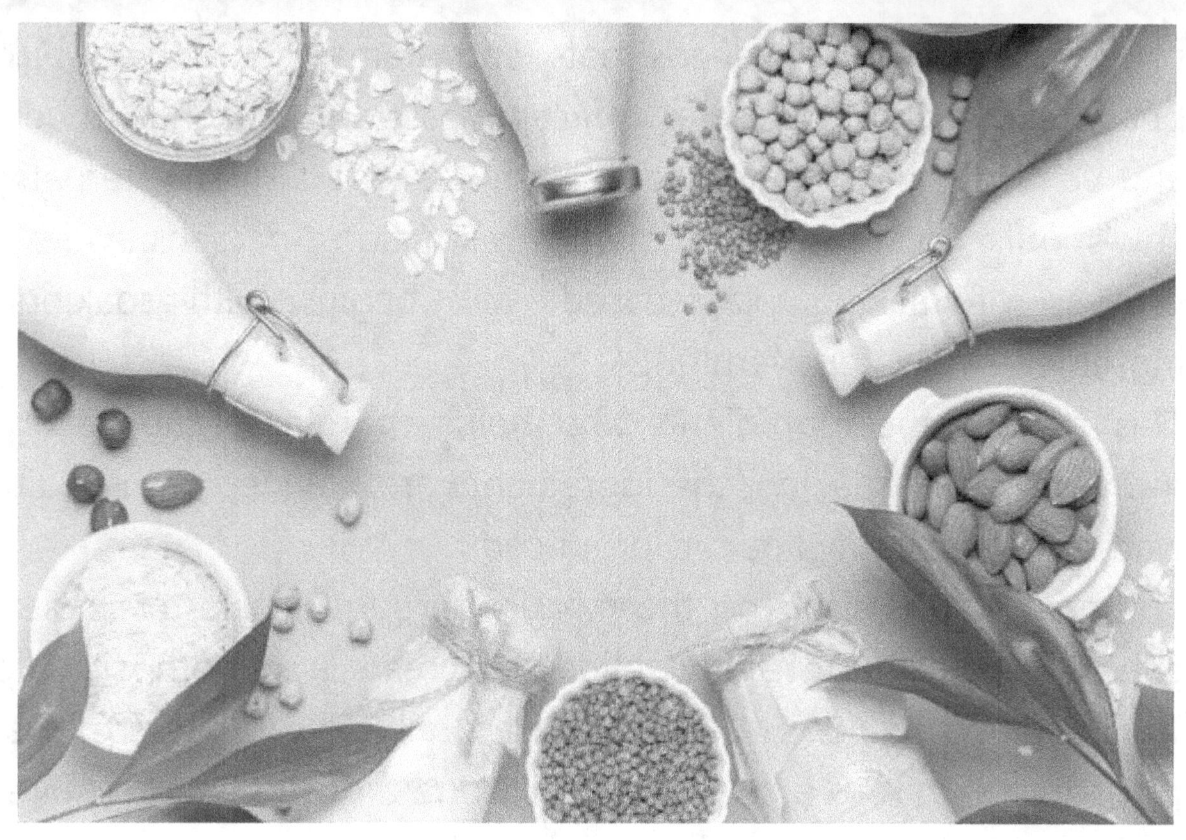

Chapter Six

Formulation and Processing of plant-based powder milk

Making plant-based milk is a relatively simple process that involves soaking, blending, and straining the ingredients. Plant-based milk, also referred to as non-dairy milk, is made from a variety of plant sources including nuts, seeds, oats, and grains. Plant-based milk has become increasingly popular in recent years due to its health benefits and versatility in cooking and baking. It is also a great alternative to cow's milk for those with dietary restrictions or sensitivities. The process of making plant-based milk begins with soaking the ingredients in water overnight.

This softens the ingredients and helps to release the flavor and nutrients. After soaking, the ingredients are blended with additional water until a creamy liquid is produced.

The next step is straining the mixture through a fine mesh sieve or cheesecloth to remove any solids and create a smooth, silky liquid. The resulting liquid is the plant-based milk. The process of making plant-based milk is a straightforward one and does not require any special equipment or ingredients. The process is also very customizable, as different ingredients can be used to create variations in flavor and texture. For example, nuts can be used to make a creamy, nutty milk, while oats and grains can produce a lighter, smoother milk. Adding sweeteners and spices can also be used to create a beverage with a unique flavor.

Generally, the process of making plant-based milk is a simple one that does not require any special equipment or ingredients.

It can be customized to fit any dietary needs or preferences and is a great way to add variety to your meals. With a little creativity, you can make delicious plant-based milk that is both nutritious and delicious.

Chapter Seven

Ingredients and Equipment

Making plant-based milk is a simple process that can be done in the comfort of your own kitchen with minimal effort and a few ingredients. To get started, you will need the right ingredients and equipment.

Ingredients needed for making plant-based milk include: nuts, seeds, legumes, grains, or other plant-based sources like coconut, oats, nuts, or soy. You will also need filtered water and a sweetener such as maple syrup, agave, or dates. Additionally, you may need additional ingredients like spices, fruits, or nut butter for flavor.

The equipment needed for making plant-based milk is fairly minimal. You will need a blender, a strainer, a container for the finished product, and a cheesecloth or nut milk bag. The blender should have a high-speed setting so that it can blend the ingredients properly. The strainer is needed for straining out any solids after the milk has been blended.

The container should be a glass jar or bottle with a tight-fitting lid. The cheesecloth or nut milk bag should be made from a fine mesh material so that you can strain out any small particles.

Once you have all the ingredients and equipment, you are ready to start making plant-based milk.

The process is fairly simple and can be done in just a few steps. First, you will need to soak the desired plant-based ingredients in water for a few hours. After that, you will need to drain and rinse the ingredients and then put them in the blender with the filtered water and sweetener.

Blend the ingredients on high until they are fully combined.

Next, strain the mixture through the cheesecloth or nut milk bag, and then pour the liquid into the container. Finally, store the finished product in the refrigerator and enjoy.

Steps

Making plant-based milk is a great way to enjoy a dairy-free alternative. Plant-based milk is made from a variety of plant-based sources such as nuts, soy, oats, and more.

There are a few steps to making plant-based milk, which include soaking the nuts or grains, blending them, and straining them. Here is a breakdown of the steps for making plant-based milk.

The first step in making plant-based milk is to soak the nuts or grains. This is important as it helps to soften and release the nutrients from the nuts or grains. The nuts and grains should be soaked for several hours, or overnight for best results.

Make sure to cover them completely with water. Once the nuts or grains are soaked, they should be drained and rinsed before being used. The next step is to blend the soaked nuts or grains.

Add the nuts or grains to a blender with 3-4 cups of water and blend until it is smooth and creamy. You can also add other ingredients such as dates, vanilla extract, or salt to enhance the flavor of the milk. Finally, the blended ingredients need to be strained.

This can be done by pouring the mixture into a fine mesh strainer or cheesecloth.

The liquid that is strained out is the plant-based milk. After straining, the plant-based milk can be stored in an airtight container in the refrigerator for up to a week.

Making plant-based milk is a simple process and can be done in just a few steps. By soaking the nuts or grains, blending them, and straining them, you can easily make a delicious and nutritious plant-based milk. Enjoy your own homemade plant-based milk.

1. Soaking

Making plant-based milk is a great way to get a wide variety of nutrients into your diet. The process is relatively simple and can be done in the comfort of your own home. The first step in the process is soaking the plant of your choice. This is done to soften the plant and make it easier to blend. The amount of time you need to soak the plant material will depend on the type of plant you are using. For example, if you are using almonds, you will need to soak them for 12-24 hours. If you are using oats, you will need to soak them for 8-12 hours. If you are using cashews, you will need to soak them for 4-6 hours. When soaking the plant material, you will want to use a ratio of 1 cup of plant material to 2-3 cups of water. Once the plant material has been soaked, you will need to drain and rinse it.

This will ensure that any excess starch or impurities are removed. After the plant material has been rinsed and drained, it is ready to be blended with fresh water.

You can use a blender, food processor, or immersion blender to blend the plant material. You will want to use a ratio of 1 cup of plant material to 3-4 cups of fresh water. This will help create a creamy, smooth milk. Once the milk has been blended, you will want to strain it using a nut milk bag or cheesecloth. This will help remove any remaining chunks of plant material. After the milk has been strained, it is ready to be enjoyed.

You can add sweeteners, spices, or other flavorings to customize the milk to your taste. Making plant-based milk is a relatively simple process that can be done in the comfort of your own home.
The first step in the process is soaking the plant material.
This is done to soften the plant and make it easier to blend. Once the plant material has been soaked, drained, and rinsed, it is ready to be blended with fresh water. After the milk has been blended and strained, it is ready to be enjoyed.

2. Blending

Making plant-based milk is a simple and nutritious way to add flavor and variety to your meals. Plant-based milks are made from a variety of nuts, grains, and even legumes. The process of making plant-based milk involves soaking, blending, and straining. The second step in the process is blending.

Blending is an important part of making plant-based milk because it breaks down the ingredients and helps to release their nutrients and flavors.

To blend plant-based milk, you'll need a blender and the ingredients that you've soaked. Start by adding your soaked ingredients, such as nuts, seeds, or grains, to the blender.

Then add some water to help the blender run smoothly and blend the ingredients until the mixture is smooth and creamy. You can also add other ingredients, such as sweeteners, spices, or flavorings, to the mixture before blending.

Once your mixture is blended, you can strain it with a cheesecloth or a nut milk bag. This will help to remove any particles or debris from the liquid. If you'd like a thinner consistency, you can add more water to the mixture and blend it again. If you'd like a thicker consistency, you can add more of the soaked ingredients before blending.

Blending is an important part of making plant-based milk, as it helps to break down the ingredients and release their flavors and nutrients. It's a simple step, but it's key to making a delicious and nutritious plant-based milk.

3. Straining

The process of making plant-based milk involves several steps. One of these steps is straining. Straining plant-based milk is the process of removing the solids from the liquid.

This step is important for achieving a smooth, creamy consistency.

The first step in straining plant-based milk is to pour the liquid into a large container or bowl. For a fine-textured milk, use a nut milk bag or cheesecloth.

Place the cloth over the container and slowly pour the milk through the cloth. This will filter out any remaining solids. Once all of the milk has been strained, the solids can be discarded.
If you are straining a thicker milk, such as oat milk, you may need to use a sieve. Pour the milk through the sieve and use a spoon to press down on the solids.
This will help separate the solids from the liquid. Once all of the milk has been strained, the solids can be discarded. When straining plant-based milk, it is important to be gentle and patient.
This will help ensure that the milk has a smooth, creamy texture. If any chunks of solids remain, they can be blended in a blender or food processor to achieve a smoother consistency. Straining plant-based milk is an important step in the process of making plant-based milk. It helps to remove any remaining solids, which is important for achieving a smooth, creamy texture.
Straining can be done using a nut milk bag or cheesecloth, or a sieve for thicker milks. With patience and care, straining can help ensure that the milk has a smooth, creamy texture.

4. Flavouring

Making plant-based milk is an easy and healthy way to enjoy a dairy-free alternative to dairy milk. Flavoring the milk is the last step in the process and is an important step for creating a delicious, unique-tasting product. There are a few different ways to flavor plant-based milk, such as adding syrups, extracts, spices, and fruits.

One popular option is to add a syrup or extract to the milk.

Syrups such as maple or agave are a great way to add sweetness to the milk, while extracts like vanilla or almond can add a unique flavor. Depending on the flavor desired, different combinations of syrups and extracts can be used to create a unique flavor.

When adding syrup or extract to the milk, it is important to start with a small amount and add more as desired. Another option for flavoring plant-based milk is to add spices. Spices such as cinnamon, nutmeg, and cardamom are great options for adding a unique flavor to the milk.

The amount of spice added will depend on the desired flavor and can be added to taste. It is important to start with a small amount of spice and add more as desired. Finally, fruits can be added to plant-based milk to create a unique flavor. Fruits such as berries, bananas, and peaches are great options for adding sweetness and flavor to the milk. When adding fruits to the milk, it is important to start with a small amount and add more as desired.

The fruits can be blended with the milk in a blender, or added to the milk after it has been heated. Flavoring plant-based milk is an easy and fun way to create a unique, delicious product.

By adding syrups, extracts, spices, or fruits to the milk, it is possible to create a variety of flavors.

It is important to start with a small amount of each ingredient and add more as desired to create the desired flavor. With a little creativity, it is possible to create a delicious plant-based milk that everyone will love.

5. Storing

Storing plant-based milk is similar to storing dairy milk. You should always store it in the refrigerator and use it within five days of opening it. Most plant-based milks are shelf stable so you can store them in the pantry unopened for long periods of time. However, once the carton is opened, you should store it in the refrigerator. When storing plant-based milk, it is important to make sure the container is securely sealed to prevent air from getting in and spoiling the milk. If you are storing it in a carton, make sure the lid is tightly sealed.

You can also use an airtight container or a sealed Mason jar to store the milk. To make sure the plant-based milk stays fresh, it is important to store it in the back of the refrigerator in a steady temperature. The front of the refrigerator can be quite cold, which can cause the milk to spoil faster. It is also a good idea to write the date on the container when you open it so you can easily keep track of when it needs to be used. If you're not going to use the plant-based milk within five days, you can freeze it. Freezing the milk can help it last for up to three months.

Make sure you freeze it in a sealed container or a Mason jar and write the date on it when you freeze it so you can easily keep track of when it needs to be used. Storing plant-based milk is an important part of making sure it stays fresh and tasty.

Once you open the carton, make sure you store it in the refrigerator in a sealed container and use it within five days. If you won't use it before then, you can freeze it and it will last for up to three months.

Tricks and Tips

Making plant-based milk is an easy way to add more variety to your diet. It can be made from a variety of plant sources such as nuts, seeds, grains, and legumes. The process of making plant-based milk is relatively simple and can be done in a few easy steps. Here are some tips and tricks to help you make the perfect plant-based milk. The first tip is to choose the right plant source. Depending on the type of milk you're making, different plants provide different textures and flavors. For example, nuts like almonds and cashews make a creamy milk, while oats or rice create a thinner milk.

Consider the flavor and texture you're looking for when choosing the right plant source. The second tip is to use filtered water. When making plant-based milk, it's important to use filtered water to eliminate any contaminants or impurities. This will help create a cleaner and better tasting milk. If you don't have access to filtered water, you can also use bottled water. The third tip is to use a blender.

A blender is the best way to create a smooth and creamy plant-based milk. Make sure to blend on a high speed for at least one minute to ensure the ingredients are thoroughly mixed.

If you don't have a blender, you can also use a food processor or a powerful hand blender. The fourth tip is to strain the milk. After blending, it's important to strain the milk to remove any solids. The easiest way to do this is by using a nut milk bag or cheesecloth.

Simply pour the blended mixture into the bag and squeeze the mixture to remove any solids. The fifth tip is to sweeten and flavor the milk.

If desired, you can add a sweetener and flavorings to the milk.

Maple syrup, agave syrup, and honey are all popular sweeteners for plant-based milk. You can also add flavorings such as cinnamon, vanilla extract, or almond extract. Making plant-based milk is a simple and easy process. With these tips and tricks, you'll be able to create the perfect plant-based milk. Enjoy!

Chapter Eight

Conclusion

Making plant-based milk is a great way to enjoy a delicious and nutritious non-dairy alternative. The process of making it is relatively simple and requires just a few ingredients and tools. The main steps involve soaking the plant-based ingredients, blending them with water, straining the mixture, and then flavoring and sweetening as desired. Depending on the type of plant-based milk being made, the process may also include boiling and simmering.

The end result of making plant-based milk is a delicious and nutrient-rich beverage that can be enjoyed hot or cold. Plant-based milk is a great choice for those looking to reduce their dairy consumption or eliminate it altogether. It can also be used as an ingredient in recipes, such as baking, smoothies, and sauces. When making plant-based milk, it's important to use high-quality ingredients and tools. This will ensure that the milk is of the highest quality and will have the best taste and texture. Additionally, it's important to follow the recipe closely and pay attention to the instructions for soaking, blending, and straining. In conclusion, making plant-based milk is a simple and rewarding process that can be enjoyed by people of all dietary preferences. With the right ingredients and tools, it's possible to create a delicious and nutritious non-dairy alternative that can be enjoyed hot or cold. Additionally, plant-based milk can be used in a variety of recipes to create delicious dishes.